# THE WIG DIARIES

## MARY LADD

———

*Drawings by*
## DON ASMUSSEN

"Congressman Mo Brooks, Do You Want Me to Die?" was originally published on May 2, 2017 on Medium

"How Going Naked to a Hot Springs Retreat Helped Me Accept My Breast Cancer Surgery Scars" was originally published on September 29, 2017 by *Health*

ISBN: 978-1-7341333-0-1 (hardcover)
ISBN: 978-1-7341333-1-8 (ebook)

Library of Congress Control Number: 2019916067

An IngramSpark title printed by Wig Industries in the United States of America

Wig Industries
490 2nd Street #200
San Francisco, CA 94107

www.maryladd.com

Illustrations by Don Asmussen
Book design by Josh Korwin

# Table of Contents

# Is This Book for You?

Getting breast cancer serves up loss of dignity, follicles, and body parts, immense pain, dry eyes, cracked skin, and oh-so-many scars—yet laughing helps. See if you've ever felt like me.

Have you said no to an invite because you fear that constipation and diarrhea may hit your guts in the same hour and worry you won't have access to a private bathroom?

Do you know way too much about lubricants because of your Sahara-like vagina? To those fools offering "use it or lose it" advice—what's so wrong with nightly cuddling with the remote, books, and/or adorable pets instead?

For the lucky post-treatment folk, do you find yourself looking for a hulking ugly gray medical building to check into, where you can ask, "What now?"—only to find that place doesn't exist?

Does your ridiculously thinning hair (or no hair) make you sad?

When you are hugged wet-noodle-style, is it obvious that your hugger thinks your cancer will jump from your body into theirs? Since cancer is obviously contagious!

Did a well-meaning someone gift you a pink-ribboned bracelet, tutu, or oven mitt—even though you already have enough breast cancer awareness to last eighteen lifetimes?

Is it hella beyond annoying to be told, "You have cancer? But you look great!"

Do you have a PhD-level understanding of parabens and toxins and worry that they are in your water bottle, makeup, detergent, and deodorant? Maybe you've given up deodorant altogether, musty pits be damned, early menopause or not.

Have you started ingesting insane amounts of flax, green tea, cruciferous vegetables, and chia to, you know, stop cancer? Even if you usually can't even afford organic lettuce.

Are you the ultimate conversation killer, since folks go awkward and quiet when you hobble-walk in the room?

While you're maybe not a stickler for gender pronouns, does it still make you sigh every time a bus driver or barista says, "Yes sir!" because you don't have any hair anywhere… on your entire body—which may attract *acomophilia* fetishists who are turned on by baldies. Come and get me, I'm bald everywhere!

When you go blank and forget what you were going to say, do you blame it on "cancer brain"? Again?!

Do people hint that if you only drank fresh lemon water every morning, and maybe cut out sugar completely, you wouldn't have gotten diagnosed?

Have you ever been dripping in sweat from side effects or damn early menopause and wanted to roll around naked on a precariously melting ice cap?

Does your blood boil when you get unwanted advice: "Ohhh, when my cousin/friend/mom had breast cancer, she didn't get that treatment you're getting… You've got this, you're a warrior!"

Did you guiltily offer your partner the chance at an open relationship, so he/she/they could have regular orgasms?

When someone offers to bring you food, do you kinda want to say, "Only if it's free-range-wild-seafood-pesticide-free-super-organic-with-absolutely-no-added-hormones"?

Is it obvious and sad to notice the way people avert their eyes to look anywhere but at you the exact moment they realize you have cancer? Since cancer is apparently contagious.

Did you get pushed out of your job in shady fashion because of how much time you took for cancer treatment?

Does it make you mad that your bras and tops don't fit quite right STILL?!? How can one breast be so much smaller than the other after all those treatments and surgeries?!

Are you always trying to figure out the calendar end date for your cancer shit even if there doesn't seem to be one?

Have you been lectured in judgey fashion on gooey cheese, caffeine, sushi, red meat, drinking booze, and other fun things? Did you respond by telling them go ahead, take adorable puppies and hot fudge ice cream sundaes, so that you have truly nothing left to live for?

When you spit in a plastic cup for eight really long minutes while a dewy-looking genetic counselor with long, natural glossy locks gave you a welcoming smile, did you want to scream?

Are you furious at refineries, frackers, and other polluters, wondering how much the environment played a role in your diagnosis?

Do people hit you up for advice on the best medibles and tinctures?

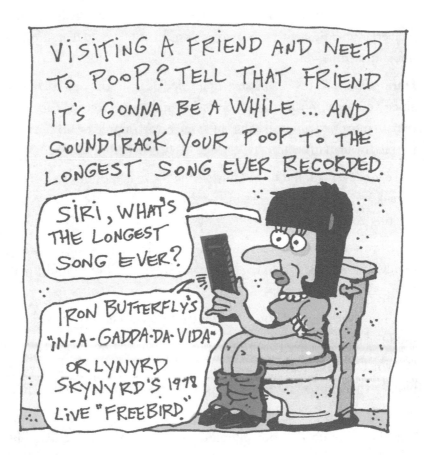

When you feel pain or tingling where your real boobs used to be, do you worry that cancer is growing and bubbling and taking over your body?

While everyone you know is asleep (annoying!), do you sit there in the dark, crying over friends who have died or are close to dying from breast cancer, as well as your own symptoms, recurrence likelihood, and the always scary medical bills?

Did you receive a ton of unwanted, ineffective "hopes and prayers" messages?

As you hobble-walk across the street, do you wish you had an "I have cancer!" sign? Since it's not anyone's dream to be honked at, flipped off, and/or run over.

During sexy time (even solo sexy time), do you insist on total darkness, since you have too many embarrassing and ugly surgery scars and remain mortified about having only one breast/nipple or no breasts/nipples instead of two?

Have you ever wanted to verbally shame the male politicians aiming to make medical care impossible for those of us who are walking pre-existing conditions?

When you screamed at your family for using the microwave, did they totally not understand how much you fear simple household items that may or may not cause cancer?

Has someone ghosted you when you got cancer because they don't want to face their own mortality?

Did you ever have the hots for the medical professional who drew your blood, wheeled you into surgery, or wiped your butt in the hospital no matter their age or gender?

When you are on hold for 147 minutes, trying to get a medical-bill question answered, do you try not to panic over being sent to collections over a $9 blood draw that got lost in your scary mountain of bills?

Last one. Does reading these FAQs, and knowing that there are humans who 1,000 percent get what your life with breast cancer is like, make you feel a teensy bit supported and possibly happy-ish? You win! And by win, I mean: this book is for you.

It makes a great bathroom reader. Patients, check that your toilet seat is as soft and cushy as possible, since you'll spend too many minutes on the toilet.

\* \* \*

*The Wig Diaries* tells the story of getting through seven cancer surgeries, eight infections, sixty-nine blood tests, one over-the-top crush on my surgeon, and twenty-two rounds of chemotherapy. I joined the ranks of the estimated 1 in 9 women to be diagnosed with breast cancer in America.

Following the brutal results of genetic testing, I decided to have both breasts removed. New breasts were formed out of my belly fat, which basically means I now have breasts made of cheese, chocolate, and bread.

The next act was a hysterectomy and the insta-menopause that made me even more dried up. I was thirty-nine.

# THE 4 STAGES OF PITCHING A CANCER HUMOR BOOK

### By Don Asmussen

People with cancer desperately need humor. Will somebody tell publishers?

## STAGE 1. DETECTION

Publishers will try to tell you that your cancer isn't funny. Don't believe them. At one point in our history, the entire country believed "Three's Company" was funny. *Nobody knows shit.*

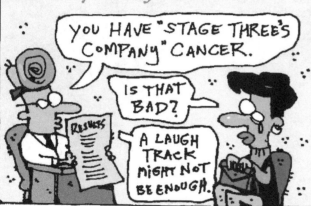

YOU HAVE "STAGE THREE'S COMPANY" CANCER.

IS THAT BAD?

A LAUGH TRACK MIGHT NOT BE ENOUGH.

RESULTS

## STAGE 2. TREATMENT

Publishers love dog books. "Marley & Me" sold like a bazillion copies. Use it as a template for a cancer book.

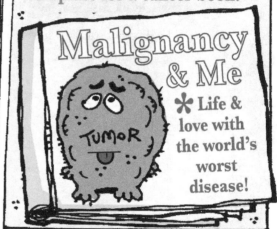

Malignancy & Me

TUMOR

\* Life & love with the world's worst disease!

## STAGE 3. PREVENTION

Publishers will tell you that cancer is "already taken" by another humorist.

### Renowned Disease Comedians

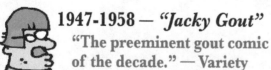

**1947-1958 — *"Jacky Gout"***
"The preeminent gout comic of the decade." — Variety

**1958 — *"Jimmy Shingles"***
"The hottest shingles comic of mid-to-late 1958." — TV Guide

**2014 - present — *"Tig Notaro"***
"She'll make you want to heckle all other cancer sufferers" — Time

## STAGE 4. RECOVERY

Publishers will finally convince you to write the erotically-charged "Four Shades of Cancer" book series and just accept God's plan (and royalties)…

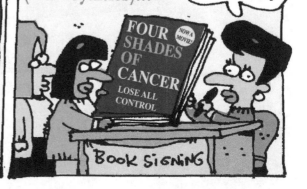

FUCK IT.

FOUR SHADES OF CANCER
NOW A MOVIE
LOSE ALL CONTROL

BOOK SIGNING

# *A Very Important Cancer Message from the Cancer Artist of this Cancer Book.*

## BY DON ASMUSSEN

Attempting to publish a humorous cancer book is a lot like having cancer.

Let me explain:

1. You send some samples to a Publishing Lab.

2. The Publishing Lab sends those samples to an off-site facility for several weeks (or months) to see if your mix of nouns, verbs, adjectives, and adverbs (also gerund levels) are normal.

3. The results come back and everything appears fine. Yet, the Publishing Lab is still hesitant.

4. Further tests reveal that your humor levels are too high, possibly due to iron deficiency.

5. Further PET scans suggest that this humor has metastasized throughout your body, making it impossible for you to be inspirational, courageous, or serious.

6. The Publishing Lab tells you to try to be more inspirational or courageous or serious, as opposed to humorous. Humor is death.

7. You try ... but you choose to accept God's plan. His/her plan is for you to be humorous.

8. The Publishing Lab sadly advises that you should prepare your family for the worst and that you should get your non-published finances in order.

9. You finally give up on all the major Publishing Labs, as they all use the same off-site facility.

10. You self-publish. The End (no, not THE end).

So that's the cycle. Mary Ladd and I have decided on "alternative" publishing, using various marijuana and dietary supplements instead of taking the cancer high road (well, marijuana is sort of taking the *high* road) in our attempt at the Henry Miller "spit in the face of cancer" model.

We get it, publishers are scared of death. Hell, *we're* scared of death.

But you know that point that you get to when you're *so* sad and *so* scared and *so* hysterical that you finally start laughing, just for the release?

No?

You don't?

Well, then read this book.

As the old-school comedian Henny Youngman once said, "Take my cancer ... please!" *(rim shot)*

# CHAPTER 1

## *My Wiggy Roots*

I like to laugh enough to have snot come out of my nose. As a tall and awkward gal, I have always turned to fashion as a shield for what's really going on with me. Talk to me about scarves or bracelets anytime! This book's essays should get you laughing, since it covers graphic and scary cancer details. You may also find yourself crying or sighing. Perhaps you'll even feel understood.

Why wigs? Why fashion? How did I get here?

I was the first child born to evangelical Christian hippies in San Francisco. Church was their everything. My parents and I lived in a small apartment in the Haight-Ashbury district, a few blocks from Golden Gate Park, a verdant oasis and home to concerts, drum circles, and exercisers of all sorts. We returned to this area often, even after moving to smaller Bay Area towns further east. Androgyny was everywhere. On those San Francisco streets, there were also freaky fashions. And a lot of older women wearing wigs and colorful frocks that offered more coverage—skirts knee length or longer. They walked slowly, using their canes or walkers. Music played day and night. Society's norms were upside down. I loved it.

From an early age, I felt drawn to all this fashion. But really, I loved the fabulous, free, and thrift-shopped. I had to. We didn't have much. But my grandmother back in West Virginia made and shipped custom beautiful dresses and outfits that turned me into a living doll. I hated getting measured by my mom. It made me fidgety.

My brother, Josh, was born thirteen months after me. There are way too many pictures of us in identical outfits picking flowers from a vacant lot and for various holidays and church gatherings.

Our eccentric Great-Aunt Madeline was a loving but infrequent presence. Maybe because she was so old. A visit to her San Francisco home put me in a daze. She answered the door wearing a black turtleneck and slacks, with a gray wig askew, her blue eyes sparkling mischievously. Madeline's wig was turned a quarter of an inch the wrong way, and sat atop her head like a nest, instead of looking more natural—to kinda sorta fool you into thinking she had real hair. She was friendly and nice, and talked so loud it seemed as if she were yelling. We later learned in our creaky Volkswagen, with Mom and Dad, that Madeline could not see or hear very well.

Josh and I would hide at Madeline's home to fend off boredom while the adults chatted. Silently, I would mime gagging and throwing up. We'd stifle our giggles to avoid being rude or worse, getting in big trouble with our parents. Madeline had forty-eight cats and was cooking steak for them. I wanted to find a cat bowl and get some of that steak. It smelled amazing. But the smell of rancid cat pee and dust was stifling—it took the edge off my salivating and hunger. There was no fresh air—for some reason, Madeline kept all the windows shut, probably to keep her feline *familia* from escaping.

Maybe Madeline was trying to put on her best. No matter what pain and life stuff was going on for her, Madeline showed up for us. I was figuring out that wigs and clothes can be a shield. They communicate a message of, "Hi, everything's fine, really!" One of the most American things one can say is "I'm OK."

Our family attended a Christian church in San Francisco called Glad Tidings, where many of the women wore wigs and ornate outfits, including hats and matching purses. I also saw many beautiful getups in our new hometown of Vallejo. There, Church on the Hill, which is in the same family as Glad Tidings, took up all of our waking hours. I was awkwardly tall, with long dark brown hair and hazel eyes. Rushing to pull up white tights and putting on a slip under my dress took time and effort every Sunday. I felt itchy. This was an obligation. But the results did look good. Our church world was ours. Anyone who was not a Christian was someone to minister to and save.

There was more finery during services. The gals and even the men of the congregation got dolled up. I didn't love the long church services and mimed more faces to entertain Josh, inevitably earning a painful pinch on my arm from Mom. Watching the flair parade including more wigs was a compelling way to pass the time. It taught me I could be unique yet fit in at the same time.

Sometimes a Sunday school teacher or older male congregant would joke about "waiting" for me. If a man would talk about how beautiful I was, Dad would share that he had a gun back at home. The adults would giggle and guffaw.

My parents loved music, even non-Christian tunes, and I would study Dad's album covers for clues into the bigger world. I would often ask him questions about the musicians. Maybe I was trying to figure out how and why they became who they were. Or even how they found their creative freedom. Record stores were another source of vinyl inspiration. I could headbang, pretend to strum a jazz guitar, and lady bop as I browsed, carefully looking at what the other browsers wore.

When MTV debuted, I would stare at images of singers and bands. Statement hair and wigs looked big and bright on Sheila E., Prince, Cyndi Lauper, Dolly Parton and Debbie Harry. The looks and locks of David Bowie, Boy George, Grace Jones, Elton John and Liberace also excited, because it was gender-bending and wrong according to my church. Yet they looked like people I wanted to be friends with. There were many similarities between the singers at my church and drag/mainstream performers. While their song material differed, putting on a pretty face and awesome duds topped by memorable locks seemed paramount. I found drama, theater, and entertainment, and the wigs, makeup, and outfits on TV and at church kept me wanting more.

Since I've been sick, I've found that taking an every-day-is-a-costume-party approach is a good way to get me out of bed (except when I have undiagnosed depression) and get through whatever shit show life deals me.

## CHAPTER 2

# *Wigging Out*

Wigs are heartening style savers for mornings when even my face and dome look naked and barren. It worries me to have no eyelashes, and eyebrow pencil points out the obvious: that my body is producing zero hair. A wig is a perk-me-up, allowing me to embrace feeling like someone else: maybe I'll be a blond, or a longhaired mermaid, or even Cleopatra since that eyebrow pencil already looks pretty obvious and striking, depending on which please-oh-please-get-me-through-this-day wig suits my mood. Although I am surprised at the way it affects me to lose my long auburn locks from being super sick, the fashion benefits from wigs boost the ego. Big-time.

When I am diagnosed with breast cancer, I start writing long emails to friends who keep sending me an innocent but annoying question: "How are you doing?"

The Wig Report, as I titled these email blasts, let me share outrageously funny and sad things happening in my life. Later, the emails evolved to the sassier, more relevant *Wig Diaries* on the advice of writer Mary Roach.

In quick fashion, I realize I have the hots for my plastic surgeon. His fancy Italian socks and sparkling eyes tempt and divert me from my own reality, which includes too-frequent discomfort and pain but also sadness and uncertainty.

A wig boosts my confidence enough that one day, I tote my own DIY cheese plate to a medical appointment, pretending to be a lady who lunches—my thrift-store clothes and bank account aren't fancy, but I am having a happy moment.

Well-meaning friends like to come up with cancer tips. Like eat more veggies. OK, but don't take away my cheese.

When I bust out the cheese plate in the waiting room, other patients give me weird looks. Maybe they want my Cowgirl Creamery butter knife? The facade and feeling of looking put together helps get me over the discomfort of having another blood test and worse.

While I slather goat cheese on some crusty bread, I ignore the drab surroundings and realize it's more fun and eccentric to upend the usual routine of waiting and waiting and waiting for my turn with doctors and medical staff.

Noshing lets me forget why I'm there for a few seconds and focus on something tasty, a tad naughty, and definitely pleasurable rather than get irritated at how long and cold my wait is. And yes, always offer the staff some cheese.

Poetry and spiritual books with glowing candles on the cover are acceptably nice gestures but do not address my reality. I need to laugh and smile, and my sense of humor turns out to be the best tool for navigating hellish phone calls with medical billers or ignoring adorable little mean girls who want me to take off my wig so they can see my bald head. That'd be a no, you little brats.

*The Wig Diaries* is my way of sharing how much cancer sucks and what it is like to say inappropriate things to medical staff, be stuck in my bathroom, and have oozing and super smelly wounds that look like thick coffee gravy from so many hospital visits.

When I completely lose my hair and eyebrows, I cheer myself by experiencing life as an Andy Warhol-style blond—when I was a teenager, I would read about Warhol and was drawn to how creative and totally odd he was. Another, longer wig is an obvious and over-the-top version, but putting it on makes me laugh, which feels like a sunny surprise, and helps me forget my sorrows for a few seconds.

Another bonus is losing thirty pounds, a process that sorta helps me at last understand why folks eat salad for lunch. Even if a salad makes me hungry 23.5 minutes later. Salad eaters still strike me as missing out on bigger and better things. I lost weight because of a preventative surgery related to this cancer—more on that soon.

Leading up to my diagnosis, I had for years happily gobbled cheese and meat and fried foods, along with multicourse meals. "For work." (I catered and planned events and was a food writer.) I still love cheese, but lost weight because well-meaning friends brought me healthier fare. The number of roasted chickens we got was pretty steep. It all made me feel better. I had more energy and felt literally lighter by eating differently. Let's be honest, though. I squealed with delight over a beautiful homemade *carnitas* offering, and enjoy meaty numbers. I just eat that sort of thing less often.

When I fantasize that Prince is playing an epic music set to me while I sweat it out on the toilet (side effect city, here I go), the overarching lesson is that yes, cancer sucks. It's terrible. Yet life can still feel like a funny party, especially when it includes mysterious handsome doctors, constipation, enemas, blood draws, and morphing medical circumstances. With a cabinet of wigs and scarves, I psych myself up to being game to experience it all.

# CHAPTER 3

## *Diagnosis*

Strangers (real estate speculators) are walking around my San Francisco apartment, their shoes squeaking and creaking as they walk across the wooden floors that are worn and stained from use and time. When I get a call from a number I don't even know, I assume it's the realtor or something related to these showings. Within a few seconds, I realize I need to go into the bedroom and close the door so I can better hear what this woman, a doctor I've never met, is saying.

The doctor has bad news. It's not pretty or good. She's using the D-word: Disease. I try to think about famous ladies who have had breast cancer. Their faces represent a diverse slice of ladyhood: Julia Louis-Dreyfuss, Christina Applegate, Joan Lunden, Judy Blume, Angelina Jolie, Hoda Kotb, Robin Roberts, Suzanne Somers, Gloria Steinem, Dame Maggie Smith, and Kylie Minogue. Their faces roll through my brain, and I will think of each of them later, when I'm lonely and scared in the middle of the night. Dr. Google is the WORST. I feel some comfort as I grasp that each is now in relatively good health.

And yet there's ringing in my ears. Maybe that's normal when learning you have a serious disease? There's also light dizziness. Holding on to the closet door until the spots go away feels wise, to avoid falls.

I run down the stairs, as I talk too fast into the phone. I am sprint-walking to a nearby parklet that has been a source of comfort and greenery—thankfully, it gets me far away from all of the whispers and stares back at the apartment. Tears are running down my face. If I saved one of my son's baby blankets, I could have for sure used it for what is turning into a HUGE crying jag.

I wonder if I need yoga breathing, even though I think it's silly. The word "disease" causes me to forget to breathe. Without knowing it, I pant like one of those small annoying dogs that people gussy up with expensive outfits and bows. Mascara and tears are all over my face.

Having a disease means I need more information ASAP. I need to form a timeline or plan that will of course morph and change and drag out. On the phone, the lady doctor offers hope, saying this all may soon be a terrible memory if (a big if) I luck out and get better.

The doctor says, "This is not what you had planned."

No shit! I am three months from turning forty. It is a sunny September day, and I had been looking forward to attending my son's back-to-school night for the first grade. I kid. I was *obligated* to attend back-to-school night.

I call my husband, Oscar, who is confused by the info I am quickly giving him on the phone. He offers to pick up our kid in an hour, and we decide to meet somewhere down the street for dinner.

I need an ice cream cone after getting this terrible and unexpected news. Who says food can't distract me from even this? I need to feel alive and cared for, and the chocolate cone will be sweet, filling, and calming—just enough to get me through the shock.

In front of a popular ice cream shop, I sit in dazed silence and wonder what caused my disease: too many beers? Maybe too many medium rare steaks or barbecued cheeseburgers? Or perhaps my love of sparkly

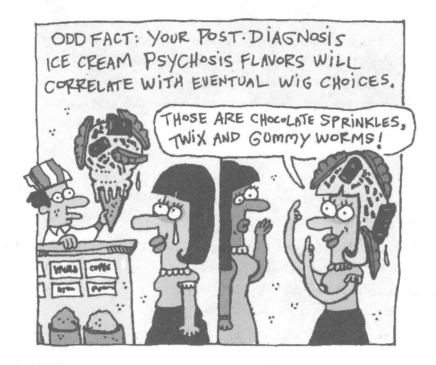

makeup is a factor—I love me some affordable drugstore beauty goodies, even if Wet n Wild sounds more like a stripper show.

In the coming weeks, when my mind wanders, I will continue to search for the reasons why I am sick, and blame thrift store furniture and the refineries that pollute the skies in my region.

The doctor had said to not go to back-to-school night. She's right, I would probably look at all those kiddos and just burst into tears, wondering how long I will be around. I don't cry while we eat dinner, but instead wonder how many more days and years I have left, tucking my hands into my pockets while I sit as a way to calm down. It's good that I have big, sassy powder-pink ($5) sunglasses as we sit at an outdoor table. There's a cheeseburger for me (comfort me now, guess I'm not *that* afraid of beef), but I barely pick at my food. Obviously, something's majorly wrong.

When I try to call a few friends, my cell phone keeps crapping out. Insider tip: have a phone charger at the ready when you are relaying cancer news over the phone. The phone sounds as if it's melting—what else could go wrong on this rotten day? I'm already starting to worry about bills, our new landlords, money, bills, our new landlords, money, repeat. My call to my friend Lora drops suddenly. When I call her back, I tell her in a teary and trembling voice, "My phone doesn't want to tell you the bad news!"

We laugh over that. It cheers me up. My nose is an overflowing snot fountain.

"We're here for you. Let us know what we can do." My wish list will soon be sleep, breakfast pastries, drinking water, and comfy pajamas.

Asking the doctor what the disease will cost when I first get that diagnosis almost causes me to faint. I'm not rich, so I also ponder how to make creative "tasteful" nude videos for YouTube to fund the cost of treatment. I hope my tech-savvier friends can help me do some public flashing—Jen Craft says she's game to film me on a beach if that's what I really want to do.

Maybe I'll use a crowd-funding site, too? Soon, I will learn that being open to accepting donations from friends is incredibly tough—it feels embarrassing, too. The money stuff makes me vulnerable, but also forces me to put aside my pride and fear. Soon after I begin chemo, it will be too tough for me to walk and shop for groceries. Carrying bags—who me? I can't. Cooking and clean up, which were routine before I was diagnosed, also seem overwhelming a lot of the time.

I use email to notify folks, and my first Wig Report conveys info to a bigger group, while giving me breathing room so I don't have to answer any questions over the phone, which can be exhausting.

Here are my tips for sharing your cancer diagnosis:

1. Be prepared for some to not accept your news.

2. People (your mom, elementary school friend, for example) may try to tell you things like "So and So had cancer and is now a marathon runner, business owner, award winning baker, champion kite surfer, etc."

3. Just politely tune out when someone says something that doesn't make a lot of sense. Or resent them for as long as you like, this is the chance to live exactly as you wish! Everyone deals with craptastic news in varying ways, right? Guarantee: cancer makes people say and do weird things.

## *Sample "I Have a Disease" Text/Email*

**Subject: Some health news**

I got some bad health news. I have *[ Insert disease here ]*. The medical team is moving fast and I will have *[ Insert awful test schedule ]*.

I feel upbeat *[ this is probably a lie. Insert the emotion of your choosing ]*. Since I will be wearing a hospital gown and/or wig, I am looking forward to pretending I am an aspiring actor/stylish person/ artsy type who lives in New York or L.A. or a *[ fill in your own fantasy dramatic figure ]*.

Please forgive that I am communicating this bad news over email/text.

~~I will have more updates by~~ _____. *[ Why make promises you can't keep? ]*

Hugs (actually, air hugs, please, since my veins are sore from all those needle pokes),

*[ Insert Name Here ]*

Your friends won't pay attention to the dates, and will keep messaging you to ask, "How are you doing?" and deeper probing questions. Remember, cancer makes people act SO needy and weird.

## CHAPTER 4

# *Hair: Going, Going, Gone!*

I feel sad losing my hair. As soon as my hair starts falling out, Oscar steps up his cleanup efforts by emptying our wastebaskets every thirty-seven minutes. In my tired-lady haze, I realize that's something of a world record for action on his part.

I'm totally NOT minding my own business. Cancer obliterates many things: sexual desire, saliva production, and tear ducts. The bodily fluids, they disappear. Yet bossy tendencies are not obliterated, and perhaps I have the urge to be bossy as a way of controlling my health (cough-hacks into shoulder and giggles—I may be a lost cause when it comes to controlling).

My husband has turned into Mr. Clean overnight. In his own way, he seems to be saying buh-bye to my hair. Is the sight of my fallen hair too much a physical reminder that I am sick? Or maybe my gobs of hair strands are a potent signal that I just may die at a youngish age from this disease? Getting rid of the hairy evidence keeps our minds from going there, maybe.

Is he also thinking of how his own mom suffered and passed away of cancer, so many years ago? I snuffle-cried about never getting to meet her when Oscar and I first started dating. Uhhhh, maybe that was the

Anchor Steam beer taking over? Thinking of all the stories I've heard about her, it seems that she could bring warmth and support and caring to my precarious health business if only she were still alive.

My hair doesn't fall out in one day. It takes over two weeks. The entire process makes me look and feel more uncomfortable. Hair is such an important way to feel like a healthy human. As it starts to go, I feel more insecure than usual.

## *The Big Day*

For a work event with thousands of guests, I forget my hat. That's a move I will regret. My scalp has so many hairless white patches on full display, something a baseball cap would hide. I feel like a Halloween ghoul and tell my friend, Philip Walker, "There are big chunks of hair coming out. I'm going to have to shave it soon. Maybe today."

I don't overshare that being on display without a cap keeps me feeling itchy and anxious.

He nods and tells me it'll look great. I can't stop thinking about how much hair is coming out. It distracts me from everything else. I sprint to a local Walgreens drugstore on my break. There, I buy the best $6 hat I see—not too tough since we're in a touristy part of San Francisco. My new cheesy SF cap defies the rule that you can't wear tourist items from your own town.

Back on the job, I track the location of every garbage can and bathroom. Quick access to these dirty and stinky places offers a different relief: a spot to hide and dump the handful-size clumps of long hair that come out whenever I tug.

There's an overwhelming urge to keep pulling, pulling, pulling on my hair. The pulling seems icky yet compelling, soothing. When I pull out clumps, the hairs make a sound like moving sand around underwater. There's an odd sensation, to pull without feeling any tenderness or pain.

I was dragged by my hair as a tween. Yanked and pulled hair usually causes tender-to-the-touch degrees of agony, warmth, and swelling.

I try pulling the hair clumps out undercover—maybe no one will notice? Stealth mode is needed for this follicle game. My eyes are hidden by glamourous giant sunglasses, which hide all puffiness. I want to be sure no one is watching, which is sort of like picking my nose at a stoplight. With booger patrol, Kleenex or hands do the trick. But since my hair is shoulder length, it's tough, maybe impossible to hide what I'm *really* doing.

Since work is slow, I ask my boss, Stephanie Nix, if I can leave a little early—something I haven't done since the mortifying days when I would wear an ill-fitting tuxedo to work as a caterer. Although I feel exhausted, long days are the norm in this line of work. I always want to be invited to work on the next event by a roving crew of pros. Some of us call ourselves carnival "carnies," because the events happen in different places for different clients, and we use a lot of gear to set up and build our event, only to have it torn down by Teamsters within hours of the event closing. It usually means dirty and dusty work. Like any good logistics professional slash carnie, I'm good at smiling and greeting guests, and anticipating their needs and wants and desires. No matter if it's the drunk ones. Or the ones who say creepy pickup lines. I actually don't want to join you for anything after work. Ew.

This is the first time I try to play the sickie card. In an office that is deeply buried in a parking garage under the street, I hug my friends and thank our lady boss for a day's work.

My legs burn underneath my pants. The sun feels so bright. I would rather take a cab but am so afraid of our family's pending and ongoing bills, so onto a BART train I go. Once I find a seat, I avoid looking at the other passengers on BART. I don't know how I look now that I've pulled out so much hair today. As I try to blink my dry eyes, I don't want to spiral into more insecurity and worry. Yet I can picture the patchy uneven way my hair now looks. It bothers me to fret over my appearance.

I text Oscar from the train, "I need to shower. And have quiet. My hair is coming out today."

The message does not go through to his man brain. Maybe he's enjoying quality video game time while I'm away? Fair enough. When I get home, I am happy to see my sister-in-law, Claudia, and show her the bald patches. She has questions and gives me the biggest hug I've ever gotten from her. It's a happy shared moment. I hope that maybe our past squabbles are forgiven. Or safely nestled in the past, anyway. For right now.

Oscar tells me our incredibly fit and attractive writer friend David Guiotto is in town and will stop by. With that, I am tempted to text him an immature "WTF?!" from our bedroom, where I am splayed out on the bed, with the shades drawn so I can get away from the heat.

The only thing I think about is: How soon can I scrub my body and shave all the hair off my head?

Losing my hair makes me feel jumpy and nervous, and I want to scratch and scrub my skin all over.

Having visitors of the hot sort only makes me feel extra antsy. David has a great smile and bikes twenty miles "for fun" and knows how to write and build things. He's totally hunky and charming, the whole package, basically. I have been itchy and scratchy for the past ten hours, and am tired of waking up to long dark hairs on my face, body, and bed. There's the added feeling of never feeling clean whenever my hair falls out in huge clumps. I know I can't be cordial. Or act normalish.

Feverish, obsessive feelings race through my tired brain. I keep coming back to the startling visual of a shiny bald head.

I go in the bathroom. The bathroom door doesn't close all the way, which adds on more stress and anxiety.

Sunlight streams through the small gray window of the small bathroom. There's activity outside: kids playing, people talking, telltale cooking noises. I run the shower.

Next, I get ready to buzz all my hair off with an electric razor. The different blade guards, which are numbered, are made of black plastic and are an eighth of an inch different, depending on how short you want to go. It seems organized and pleasingly streamlined: pick a length, snap the blade guard on the top of the razor, and let the hair fly.

This razor has been collecting dust in a closet overstuffed with toilet paper rolls, bath towels, and cleaning supplies. When my son, Cipriano, needed a haircut, I used the razor a few times to save money, a theme I've followed most of my life but especially after parenthood.

When I once botched Cipriano's haircut so badly, it was definitely not the cool-kid preschool vibe I was going for. The two missing bright, white squares showed on Cipriano's scalp and his bangs were crooked. Oscar pleaded for me to just shell out money for a real haircut by professionals. Hair detectives: you can always spot a bad hairdo by the telltale baseball cap, and perhaps hunched shoulders. I asked Cip in a sing-song voice to please keep the cap on until we could get him to a proper haircut.

In the bathroom, I buzz and watch the threads and clumps of hair fall away. Think how hot Natalie Portman was when she shaved her head for *V for Vendetta*. Other hotties with shorter hair come to mind: Sinead O'Connor, Grace Jones, Amber Rose, Jada Pinkett Smith, Lady Gaga, Shannon Doherty, and Sharon Stone. I try to cheer myself up, thinking, "If they can pull it off, maybe I can, too."

It's tough—I want to distract myself yet feel a little sad and uncertain. The wastebasket overflows with my long locks. In the mirror, the bags under my eyes seem bigger than usual. On the good side, the eyes look bright. Maybe I can force myself to try to feel a little bit hopeful about the ways I can use this new look.

Seeing my bald head makes me stand up taller, but I still am not ready to share this new look. I pull my shirt down to look at the slash on my chest, where the doctors installed my port—it allows the chemo nurses to plug an IV in right through my skin. I like looking at the slash.

I pretend that I am a sexy and tough robot, who is not capable of going outside the bathroom until Hottie David leaves our place with Oscar. I'm happy Oscar has a way to get out of the house and get away from my disease and the bills and uncertainty it brings, but I wish the visit from David could have been better timed.

Once the hair is fully gone, I start to feel a further sense of loss. My hair is me. It's who I am. As a teen, whoa, did I spend a lot of hours teasing and curling it, sealing it all with gallons of Aqua Net hairspray. Now, losing the physical hair is yet another thing to mourn and feel wistful about.

In the following weeks and months, I will feel a pang of sadness whenever I come across long hairs in our apartment. They're still on my clothes. Each long hair is a reminder of what I used to be. Long hair symbolizes life before I was sick. Before I knew I'd have to have surgeries, so many blood draws, and treatments. Deep down, I know that my hair is not really a source of mental strength, but sometimes I feel guilty and vain for missing having all my hair. Aren't there bigger concerns to spend my time on? Exhibit A: medical bills.

## CHAPTER 5

# *Wig Time*

Months before I was diagnosed, I bought a wig and decided to try it out for a special date night. When my husband saw me in a jewel-colored blue dress with a long red wig on, he told me, "You look like a prostitute."

I thought I looked like a curvy 1950s movie siren. Or a gussied-up version of maybe the Little Mermaid, if she had a hot auntie?

Cipriano told me I was a witch. Oops!

That first wig is not subtle, and the length and shade of hair probably too crayon-red bright to look normal and real. With any wig, I want to look like a more exciting version of myself, but after receiving those witch/hooker comments, I stow the wig messily in a cabinet without wearing it outside.

Fast-forward to having cancer. Although most women wear wigs for nine to twelve months when they are ill, fun and saucy informative tips on buying and caring for wigs are scant. I at first feel cautious about wearing a wig. Yet the idea of getting a stable of wigs helps me pretend that I am a mermaid, Beyoncé, Andy Warhol, or Elizabeth Taylor—maybe all of the above.

Shopping for a wig indulges my inner drag queen while literally making me hotter. Like sweaty-hot.

Maybe I seek a spring in my step because cancer makes me so, so, so tired. It's depressing. I shop for a wig as a treat when I wake up groggy from a two-hour port surgery, by which a tube is attached to the right side of my chest. The port is billed as a helpful way to take the bee-sting feel out of chemo and blood pricks. It's important to build fun distractions. That means telling myself sure, I can read all the trashy gossip I want in the doctor's office.

Celeb gossip jazzes up those earth-tone rooms often filled with pale, raspy, and rickety patients.

The wig shopping request confuses Oscar. He asks, "Shouldn't we go home so that you can rest?"

That's no way to talk to a pushy patient who knows what she wants. I need to do this. Now.

"My hair is falling out!" Exhibit A: repulsive handfuls of hair in our shower drain.

I feel so afraid and sad and mad at what I see in the mirror. Losing hair and being bald pushes my insecurity buttons, too, because I don't look normal or feminine or like myself. Or what I will soon come to think of as "pre-cancer" me.

Chris Wilhite and her crew at San Francisco's Friend-to-Friend shop for sick patients help. I love that Chris has had cancer and knows my friends Amy Callaway and Barbara Denson. Chris seems to know my pain and what I'm going through.

A darker wig doesn't feel as fun, even though it's close to my usual hair color. In my buzzy exhausted state, I home in on a short blond number. Oscar says, "Blond? Are you sure?" to each blond selection, and isn't smiling.

The staff members do not cringe when I try on various blond wigs—none of them are trying to talk me out of anything my little sad heart desires. The women offer pleasing comments for one particular wig. I want to roll my eyes at the man in the room.

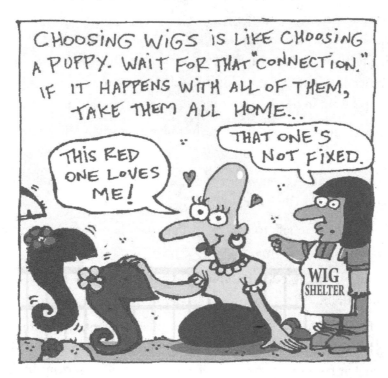

"Wow, it really suits you," one of the staffers offers, as I look at myself in the mirror, feeling puffy and drained yet intrigued.

Maybe the bright colors of the shop give me courage: the space is full of colorful long scarves, caps, and related accessories. It all looks so fashiony, and I remember that I currently need and prefer comfy pants and stretchy tops. Yet, maybe some pops of color would be a good idea.

Money is on my mind. I have so many bills. The shop will give me one wig for free. I don't think I'd be here without that important factor—Momma doesn't have extra dollars for anything. Debating how and whether to take any time off work while juggling a mountain of medical debt are common issues for patients like me.

While I browse, I forget that my body hurts and my brain is foggy. Instead of feeling sad about the cancerous rock in my breast, the blond wig gives me something to look forward to. It's new and fresh. Not scary and overwhelming. Maybe, just for a bit, it's my new normal.

Soon, I enjoy appreciative looks on the street as I sport my blond look. Hey, everyone, I wore this same dress last month and you didn't notice!

## CHAPTER 6

# Treatment Time: Can You Say Yawn?

Chemo makes me thirsty and tired. Chemicals work to rid my body of cancer. But they also kill my body in so many ways. Gone is my ability to stand up straight easily, walk at my usual quick pace, or hold conversation.

Kind offers are in for rides to and from treatment, as well as offers to sit with me at chemo to keep me company. I want to be alone in the pretty chemo room and have things to myself. The rooms for chemo remind me of a spa and are not drab, sad, and depressing like what I've seen on TV and in movies. Because the offices tend to have a steady supply of fashion and gossip magazines, I'm able to indulge and check out what reality stars are doing and zone out. I miss *Time* magazine. But my brain can't read and comprehend in the same way.

When I'm in the waiting room for treatment, I'm usually happy to be a little bit chubby since the others getting treated look frail, pale, and downright rickety. I do get jealous that the office is on the same floor as a sports medicine clinic, where I imagine fit glamazons get treated for tennis injuries on their tan limbs.

There is a high occurrence of tropical fish tanks in waiting rooms, which provide ambient noise and something to gaze at when I don't want to gawk at fellow patients who seem to be much older than I am and often of the grumpy sort. I use these long stretches to do mental penance for accidentally offing a fleet of fishies when a college love left them in my care. Those dead fish may have factored in one of our many breakups, and the college love never seemed to believe me that the power went out while I was at work, something I could not control. Still, Fish Wrangler will never be a fitting title for me. What can I say?

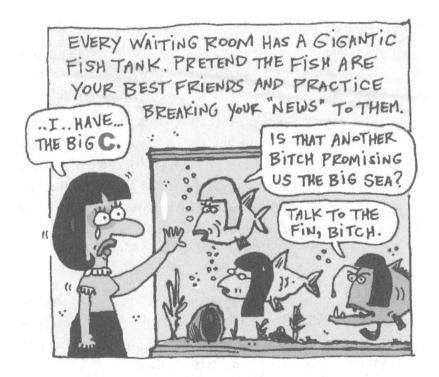

# CHAPTER 7

## *Feeling It at Walgreens*

I'm sitting down on the ground at Walgreens while my son runs around, asking me to buy him toys. There are six people ahead of me in line, and all of the four seats are filled with mortals who may need to sit more than I: canes, white hair, overweight, all of the above.

Each person in front of me seems to need a consult with the pharmacist to find out how to take their medicine, what the side effects are, and so on. It's hot and my lips and mouth are so dry. Ridiculously, the Walgreens has a bathroom that is not open to the public. Do they not see us as we wait for up to an hour? A cheery youthful staffer offers that I can buy a bottle of water instead. Plastic gives me cancer, lady! I give her a quick, "Ahhhhhh, no!" and almost put my hand in the air, oh-no-she-didn't style.

I wish my doctor had called the prescription in when I was at chemo, although he and I didn't count on my feeling nauseous and exhausted. I don't care that I'm sitting on the ground and probably picking up germs all over my hands. I am so tired these days that I can't walk up the three flights of stairs at my son's school. Standing for more than ten minutes makes me grimace and wish for my bed and dark bedroom.

I start to touch the left side of my body, to see if the tumor is getting smaller, which is sort of like masturbating in public. I am twitchy and can't help but brush the outside of my breast and push in a little bit, trying to find that rock of disease. Feeling myself up in public will turn out to be an anxious tick. It's something I do whenever I feel guilty about being grumpy to my husband and son. The wandering hands also pop up when my frazzled brain debates how soon I will be better versus the need to write my friends and family goodbye letters in preparation for dying.

## *Mannequin Inspired*

Years ago, I cooked in the home of a woman who had a mannequin she named Lady Lillian. You could not call the mannequin Lillian, she was *Lady* Lillian and propped up in a chair, all thin and beautiful. Lady Lillian sometimes sat gazing at me while I cooked with ingredients that I schlepped from Safeway, Rainbow Co-op, and the farmers' market. As I'd make batches of corn-cilantro-bell-pepper salad, salmon cakes, and eggy frittata, I sort of tried to ignore that there was a mannequin in the room. Lady Lillian got monthly costume changes that I would note in my twice weekly shifts: boho hippie with scarves, dramatic 1940s glam queen, 1980s wearer of lace and big hair.

Sometimes I feel like the cancer "journey" has gotten me to take a Lady Lillian-like approach to dressing. Lady Lillian wore different wigs, so she looked like a different lady often—something I can aspire to. I am addicted to creating looks that are so different from what I looked like before I was diagnosed. I guess everyone wants to be seen and heard in their own way, and I have never been particularly shy. But things feel markedly different: I relish diving into the free bags of clothes that dot the sidewalks and stoops of San Francisco or racking up massive $28 bills at Thrift Town, which is the mothership for Lady Lillian-style gear.

I love that things are organized by size here, a big accomplishment for any thrift operation. In my quest for redoing my look, I have ditched Hanes Her Way comfortable and high-waisted cotton panties in favor of fluorescent lacy thongs from the junior section at Target. I wish I could have ditched those comfy cotton panties one hour after a pack of boys made fun of me while I waited for a BART train, singing out to me and laughing, "Hanes Her Way! Hanes Her Way!" because the top band of my underwear was peeking out from the back of my jeans while I sat, totally unaware. My face flushed when I realized what was happening. I barked at them, pulling my shirt down to cover the flesh and underwear evidence.

I can change what my hair and clothes look like, and am genuinely happy to have eyebrows and eyelashes again. But I can't change the pretty big laundry list of internal and physical changes and pain I've been through so far. Including but not limited to:

1. Being a Bloody Valentine. In the month of October, not fair. Although ironically, this Bloody Valentine shouldn't experience vaginal penetration for another 3.5 weeks. My hysterectomy this month gifts me varying quantities of blood, a surprise-in-my-*chonies* every other time I go to the bathroom. Then there are long pauses that last for days, where I don't have to wipe, wipe, wipe away light drops of blood again.

   It's my fault for being surprised that a surgery that took out two cyst-laden ovaries and other lady parts would yield liquid that sometimes looks like fruit punch, dark Cabernet, or bright red pizza sauce.

   Food sort of repulses me these days because it makes me queasy, but food is never ever far from my thoughts.

   As long as I don't soak an entire maxipad in a short amount of time, I am healing as I should, according to my nurse. Some spotting is OK, because ten to fourteen days after a hysterectomy, it is expected for stitches to fall out from deep inside my body—maybe near where the elusive G-spot is? New cells are creating themselves, and I get to see the bloody physical results on toilet paper.

2.  Chopsticks in my belly button: I could only squint and turn my eyes to the right wall last week as the nurse put what looked like chopsticks into my belly button and began pushing and digging. "Is your belly button an innie or an outie?" she asked, while I tried to breathe like yoga people do. It looked like the chopsticks were at least three inches into my belly button. Pause. "I have no idea," I said with a tight laugh—because I could not think through the discomfort of having her tunnel deep into my belly button to "make sure everything was OK." The chopsticky thing happened after she had put a cold scope up my vagina for a few minutes to tunnel through, look at cells, and confirm things "looked good." She warned me there would be pressure on my abdomen and vagina, and sure enough, it felt just like my annual Pap smear. Thought to self: I am so looking forward to a steamy bowl of aromatic beef pho on Clement Street with my brother-in-law Steve as a reward for this digging and tunneling. It's not like I will talk about my eviscerated belly button and vag. Wrong place, wrong time.

3.  Meet my pert stomach boobs. Go ahead and stare. I am proud of these breastly beauties and haven't been this svelte since I was eight years old. Perhaps the only nice pick-me-up from my health shit storm is nabbing a smaller, tighter, perkier chest that is made out of my belly fat. All evidence of belly bulge from daily food indulgences has disappeared. I no longer need pants with drawstrings for comfort and ease, although if it's Saturday and there's a couch available, we should talk.

    I have six-pack abs and did not have to jump and sweat over any tire courses or do lunges at crazy early morning boot camps that I hear about and have zilcho interest in or money for. Since my old garb swims on me, I need new threads for my leaner and trimmer shape. Bonus if it's tight and bright. [AUTHOR'S NOTE: those six-pack abs eventually resumed their doughy form. All good.]

4. Spiderweb: My belly and groin feel as if a spiderweb is holding the cells together under my skin. When the nurse was tunneling my stomach and vagina last week, I was grateful for the spiderweb. I am sure the Spider Man connection is tied into the amount of toys and gear Cipriano collects—at one point, we would pretend to shoot spiderwebs at each other on an hourly basis. There's pain in the spiderweb region sometimes—maybe a hot slash or dull ache in one small area. Usually, the spiderweb feels like a wall that protects whatever soft material is underneath.

I also had a double enema party. Like most things in life, the mental wondering was far worse than the reality. I did almost chicken out on doing the enemas myself and called my doctor's office with semi-frantic pleas, "Are you sure I can't do a pill thing for the enema? I read about it online. Oh, OK, you're sure none of his patients does the pill instead of an enema? OK. Yes, my surgery is tomorrow."

Then I left a message for TMI, the colonic place up the street. "Do you guys take insurance? I don't think you do. Can you call me back if you do? I need to visit this afternoon, for a surgery tomorrow."

When I did the enemas at home, I was more afraid of a mouse jumping on my naked feet or butt, since we had mouse droppings show up the day before and it seemed like everywhere I looked, I saw more mice turds. It's probably a blessing to fret over mice instead of the actual pain and details of my surgery—usually I can't sleep before a procedure because I am anxious and worried. While I try to heed the call of rest and relax post-surgery (impossible), it

is really really tough to try to do that with my mousey pals around.
At least I've got some Lady Lillian scarves to put away!

## CHAPTER 8

# *Bathroom Issues (I Feel Like Shit)*

Having diarrhea one day and it-hurts-to-go constipation the next and the next feels shameful. It's definitely not something to share when anyone asks, "How are you feeling?"

I am frustrated to lose complete control of my bowels. It's as if I can't make it to the bathroom in time for an explosion of brown. Or I have to sit in the bathroom waiting endlessly.

I thought my days of cleaning up poop were long over. But here I sit, constipated and in pain in our one small apartment bathroom. I decide to rev up the internet late one night, to scan legit health websites for advice and info. I hate the dull headache that usually shows up and stays what feels like forever with constipation. Suddenly, I remember feeling mesmerized and grossed out by the *Being Bobby Brown* reality TV episode where Bobby Brown shared that he had to at one time pull poop out of Whitney Houston's butt because her turd was too big. This is gross yet helpful news I never thought I could use. More research scanning helps me figure out that I can do the same extraction instead of feeling antsy and uncomfortable for the night.

Disposable gloves and olive oil are my tools as I quietly set up in the bright bathroom. I try not to think about what I am doing with these disposable gloves. It feels like a dirty task, and I wonder more than once how much lathering and scrubbing in the shower it will take for me to feel clean.

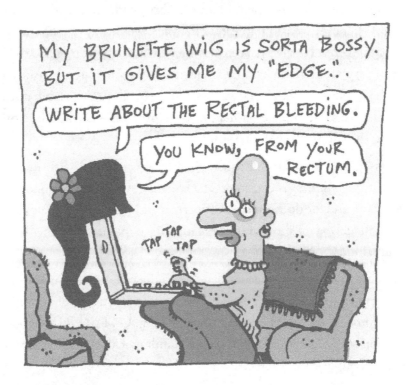

On the throne, I look down and see brown pebble-turds that fall out one at a time. I've got a goat or llama poop scene unfolding, no way does this look human. There's also a stream of bright red blood in the toilet that looks like fresh pasta sauce. I wonder if any of this will create a problem with my rectum or bowels down the line. Maybe I am tearing or scratching things and causing damage? Still, it's a heckuva lot easier to lube up the glove and remove the rocks instead of sitting with constipation for torturous stretches of up to five days. Half the battle of constipation, besides the headaches, is resisting the urge to confide in people, "I haven't pooped in three days," which would entertain my son but nah, let's not go there.

I get in touch with TT, a gay friend who teaches How to Fuck Better classes to men. TT is beautiful and healthy, with clear and healthy skin. Whenever we run into each other, his eyes always look vibrant and appealing. He always seems to be stocking up on huge bags of green vegetables. In my mind, I've decided that someone who eats so many veggies is probably regular. And since his line of work includes teaching classes on male-on-male sex, he probably has fab ideas on taking care of the back door, right?

I message: "I have an odd question but you can roll with it, I'm guessing. My illness is causing rectal bleeding when I try to go to the bathroom and the doc is not too concerned and recommends Tucks or Metamucil. Do you know of any homeopathic or natural remedies—oil, cream, foods…?"

Mr. How to Fuck Better recommends what he calls "magical foods in the form of green smoothies—soupy concoctions made of avocado, kale, spinach, etc.," to help get things moving. Or, I should try good witch hazel from Whole Foods or the Rainbow Co-op as well as sitz baths a couple times a day.

I am grateful for his advice. But, I still want dishier info from Mr. How to Fuck Better. Sitz baths are not sexy since I think of it as something for a senior citizen would need. They also remind me of advice when I was pregnant years ago: if you're constipated, take a sitz bath. Repeat. When hemorrhoids spread, do a sitz bath. I had hoped TT would read my mind regarding how to poop, with the added bonus of helping me understand how he helps people get pleasure from that back door area.

There's no way I want to share any of this with Oscar. I'd like to pretend that he doesn't know I poop. Also, what if he tells me that scratching and digging things out of myself is not a great idea? No matter if he's right. I don't want him to wonder about what I'm doing in the bathroom. Or get an idea that I am grunting and sweating on the toilet, eyes bulged out in agony. That seems like another way to put the kibosh on any potential loving, right?

Since I don't want to add to my health worries, I eventually decide it's best to let my butt do its own work, even if it's boring and frustrating to sit for soooo long. It would be weird to come out of cancer with a new, awkward-to-explain bathroom addiction. Yet if I ever again need them, disposable gloves and oil are tools for any dire situations.

# CHAPTER 9

## *ER Twilight Zone*

Is this place in network? Probably not, but that's what I get at 3 a.m. Bad lighting, apathetic door staff, and the bizarre use of paper towels instead of medical forms create more exhaustion and anxiety. How many minutes will it take me to find out what's wrong?

How much will this all cost?

I'm at the front door of the emergency room on the last day of a holiday weekend. Wondering why medical emergencies always happen during the middle of the night, when a medical visit will cost more and the chance of potentially seeing a lot of blood and guts or other drama in the waiting room beckons.

Behind the doors, there's a tall young security guard wearing a white shirt and black tie. He's chatting with someone I can't see. While he's smiling and talking away, I can tell he's ignoring me. I am waving and wiping tears off my face. Maybe that makes me look crazy. Or homeless. Maybe he's like the bouncers at nightclubs, showing his power. Could be that he's not as customer service oriented.

"I need to get in!" I say—exaggerating the words, so that he can read my lips through the glass.

He stops his chatter and shrugs a little. Then he pauses, which makes me start to feel more angry and agitated. There's a sign that says this door is not in use during late-night hours. I don't care. I need in and am starting to hunch over in pain. I am trying to manipulate him to jump up and get me to a doctor.

"How do I get in?" I ask.

He stands up and points around the corner. Shit. I'm going to have to walk around the high-rise building. I turn away in a huff. It's past 2:30 in the morning. As I turn away from the men and their chat-fest, I start mumbling "I hate you!" over and over again.

I am sad and mad that this is happening and am frustrated to be in so much pain. The city seems like it's asleep. No 49 or 14 MUNI busses in sight. No drunkards stumbling around. Definitely no cars in motion.

I want to be asleep instead of wandering around the outskirts of a giant industrial-looking building. I can hear my steps, and know that I am shuffling and bending my body from the pain. It's sort of Frankenstein-style moving, all bent and awkward. Seeing monsters in movies is both thrilling and horrifying, but I am getting scared from worrying about what is causing me to bend and hobble and how will I pay the bills for a middle-of-the-night visit. Three to six bills are almost guaranteed for this sort of hospital visit, and that's with my semi-decent insurance coverage.

The way my body moves means that something is terribly wrong. A hospital is the only place I should be with these monster moves, since it is so different from the way any lady aspiring to be healthy and normal should look and act.

Oscar wanted me to take a cab. But this hospital is around the corner from where we live. Four blocks. A third of a mile. Sitting in a cab would hurt more than walking. I also did not want to have to talk or worse, listen to any other human talk.

It's cold and I can see my breath. My side feels tender and bruised on the right, and I have cramps in my privates that jolted me from my sleep. The cramps are more severe than menstrual cramping, and since I officially don't have periods anymore thanks to early menopause, I wonder what ailment this could be.

I continue saying "I hate you!" as I walk around the building.

I walk up the ramp and am startled at the bright lights above me. I stop mumbling "I hate you" and start yawning. I'm still bent at a funny angle, and shuffle up to a different security guard to check in. "I need to see a doctor. I'm in pain," I say, dragging the last word out because I can't help myself and want to hurry up this process. He points me around the corner and says a nurse will be with me.

Inside the waiting room (awful lighting, of course), a comedy show on the TV with a music number revolving around sex offenders only adds to the confusion. I am fascinated that such a bizarre show is playing in such a public space. This is different than watching news, talk shows, or informercials, the usual waiting room entertainment options. On the other hand, seeing anything about Snuggies (wearable blanket fashion), Ginsu knives "Carve yourself a piece of the American dream," or the masturbatory-appearing Shake Weight for Men ("Increase your upper-body muscle activity by up to 300 percent") could distract in a guilty pleasure kind of way.

Minutes later, a nurse starts asking me questions. She has pretty pink nails. I am starting to wonder, though, because she's writing her notes down on a brown paper towel. Where are the billions of forms? Or charts? I would be happier with a real piece of notebook paper. The paper towel thing is bonkers, but she asks the normal questions about how long I've been in pain, is anyone at home hurting me (does Bobby Browning myself count?), have I had surgeries or other medical complications. Then, she flips the paper towel over and writes more notes on the back. Her writing looks neat enough and she's capturing the info.

Normally, I would speak up to ask why she's using a paper towel. But I can't slow things down with questions. Keeping my thoughts to myself means I'll get help soon.

When I leave the hospital hours later, I've learned that my urinary tract was *this close* to some sort of bizarre and severe bacterial vaginosis. Which explains the itching, bubbling, and suffering!

When the mail delivers bills totaling almost $2,000, it makes me wish I had opted for toughing it out or guzzling cranberry juice (I assume since it works for urinary tract infections, it would also work for severe vaginosis). But what if by not going I got a too-terrible infection or died?

# CHAPTER 10

## *Skin and Transference*

I get used to showing skin at medical appointments and shrug if a staff member walks in while I am putting on a medical gown. I wonder if years ago, maybe I should have hit amateur night at a strip club, where my friend worked when we were in our twenties. That could've slayed my credit card debt, right? Which of course leads to wondering if I could now be some sort of cancer webcam gal, flashing my slashed up bodily goods for twenty minutes a day to in turn slay my medical debt. Hmmmm.

Similarly, acting flirty with the medical team—especially if under the influence of meds—is a guaranteed way to make the staff uncomfortable. Nurses and technicians. Male or female. Anyone who wipes my butt. Or takes a cool washcloth to my forehead when I'm sweaty and crying. Maybe I'm pansexual. When I visit my favorite surgeon, I act like this is not just a medical appointment. It's the chance to be around hot folks! I'm flushed from all my treatments and am sort of faking it until I make it. The heat I feel is mainly from medically induced hot flashes, but maybe I want to eventually feel less withered and depressed.

I develop a teensy crush on my doctor the first time I disrobe and show him my bare-naked chest, arms, and stomach. He's married. I'm married. I don't care! This condition, known as transference, is my chance to indulge a fantasy without many consequences. Maybe I was primed for it by watching soap operas in junior high, or when I kept dialing the super expensive 976 romance hotline in sixth grade—Press 1 to continue your hot and steamy thoughts, girlie! Symptoms of pining for my doc include giggling and singing to myself in the shower on appointment days. This is a fabulous distraction from medical bills, rent, work, and my actual relationship. Focusing on the doctor is a fun fantasy, and I forget for a few seconds or minutes that I feel so physically weak.

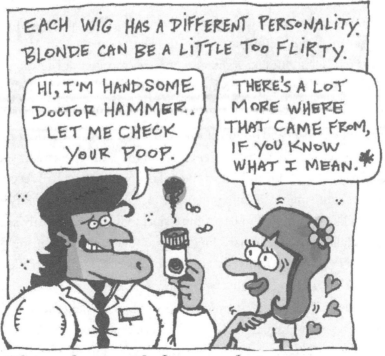

*He's a doctor, He knows what you mean.

I definitely highlight my cheeks and eyes for these doctor visits, and opt for clean and sexy non-cotton underwear. I wonder if I am crazy for wanting to check in for a surgery by myself so I can carve out some alone time with Le Doc. His eyes are friendly and sparkling. He never checks sports stats or email when I have an appointment. Probably the most compelling part is that I have never ever seen the Doc with his cellie. Just a clipboard and pen to take notes on me, me, me.

He patiently smiles and nods when I ask questions, and has such a great bedside manner. More than once, I wonder what it would be like to be in an actual bed with him. Do keep the white medical lab coat on, pretty please! My body has been so prodded and traumatized; scars on my chest and arms paired with an ongoing major dose of the sleepies help me rationalize avoiding sex back at home. Reassurance from an older, handsome man in a professional and controlled setting surprises and soothes while letting me enjoy his calm/fun demeanor. We share no heated cell phone text arguments or in-person stressful fighting. He asks me in a non-rushed way how I feel and how I'm doing. I almost bat my lashless eyes, which seems like a vain attempt to feel pretty.

In his white jacket and button-down shirt, I can cling to the idea of him as an archetype when I'm feeling blue. Surgeries and procedures that are physically painful and sometimes take months (years?) of recovery can be slightly pleasant since it involves his healing handiwork. When he acts like he thinks I'm beautiful, I start to feel it. Especially as my hair is falling out and I have huge bags under my eyes. During one surgery, I gush to two nurses, "He's soooo good-looking!" Thankfully, he's not around to hear this overshare. The nurses give me a knowing smile that shows they are used to patients on pain meds saying and doing semi-crazy things. I'll soon learn that the doctor has many adoring fans like me, who develop a crush on him for his kind and caring medical ways. I don't like the idea of being in a group of fans. Move aside, ladies and gents, and yes he has male fans. However, I do feel comforted by the fact that I am not the only one to harbor such not-so-odd fantasies.

## Surgery Makes Me Horny

Surgery makes me horny because I am showing so much skin and lying in a bed 24/7 with just a thin gown on. It's not just the chance to be examined by my Doc or the meds talking. Getting undivided attention from nurses, doctors, technicians, and of course the billing staff lets me feel like my pre-cancer self. The staff is trained to be nice to me; what a turn on! They approach and ask in soft tones about my symptoms, medications, diet, aches and pains. I used to be the one in charge of my schedule, but during surgery, I have to lie around a ton and let others do the actual heavy lifting, slicing, and dosing. Bring it.

I feel like a temptress flashing my skin to so many folks—keep in mind that I was a rebel raised by evangelical Christians. As a child, I was drawn toward dramatic and eccentric people.

My body is still hot from all the chemo, meds, and overnight menopause. Wearing a Bair Paws suit provides a spa-like experience of blasts of hot air from a suit that makes me feel like an interesting and accomplished astronaut. It reminds me of being in a pedicure chair, which I haven't done in years (time, money). This suit comes with a remote that lets me press buttons to feel different sensations. Some awesome sex toys have remotes, too.

Perhaps the most freeing part of surgery is the ability to fall asleep in a hospital bed and have the kind of rest that is dark and without any sort of worry-filled dreams. Trusting in the staff that I have flashed helps me eventually believe that my body is being taken care of. Maybe it is. Maybe not. The only thing on my to-do list is sleeping, which I am often too anxious to do. I'm also waiting to see what my new tits and body will look like.

## *What Am I Saying? It's the Anesthesia, Dear*

Dear hospital staffers, I'm sorry for telling you about a drag song called "Dildos Are Forever" right before I passed out. If you could see the extraordinary drag artist Jackie Beat sing this one at a condom couture nonprofit fundraising event, you'd become a fan, too. And I also apologize for using an offensive sing-songy voice to tell the Korean anesthesiologist "I want to go to Japan!" when he asked where I'd like to travel to next.

Male friends tell me in whispered tones that they have also confided crazy things in the operating room. One grandly announced to a packed medical house: "I like fucking!" before going under the knife for a vasectomy. Another announced in an unintentionally loud voice that "pussy popsicles" are a favorite flavor, although the diligent and likely heard-it-all nurse was offering lime or cherry.

I know the medical staff tends to be professional, and after the dildo overshare, I decide to email my favorite surgeon and apologize for creating such a hostile work environment for his team. The next time I see him in his office, he smiles and assures me that I shouldn't worry at all, with the enticing promise that I have no idea what they talk about while patients are out—my statement is not the wildest thing they've ever been subjected to. Still, my face gets redder as I fret over the details of what else I might have divulged while under the influence of anesthesia.

## CHAPTER 11

# *My Catheter Sounds Like a Waterfall*

In the hospital, I wish I could check my control issues at the door. These things really bother me while I stay in the hospital. I can't say I've ever been waterboarded or attacked by an army of red ants, but I have experienced mental and physical torture in the form of:

I can't drink water for the next twenty-four hours. While the nurse is standing over me as I wake up from surgery, sucking from her pink water bottle, I beg for water. Then beg again. I can hear her slurping from her jug and feel so thirsty, tired, and sad to not be able to put water or a teensy ice chip or three in my mouth.

I'm lying on a bed with rubber sheets, dripping in sweat. I can feel the sweat in every nook and cranny and am stuck in my own utterly uncomfortable sweat-lodge-for-one. Swishing back and forth on the bed from all the sweat and dampness makes me more crazy. I decide this may be one of the toughest nights of my life, both mentally and physically.

The sound of a trickling waterfall may be soothing to visitors, but it's my catheter causing major pressure on my innards. It feels like there is a baby crab inside me, pinching and pushing down on my bladder.

Without a release, the discomfort builds and of course I start sweating again. I'll later learn that this is not normal and I should have spoken up immediately to get the catheter adjusted. I thought extreme discomfort was par for the post-op course, Doc. Do I win a prize for being a martyr? No. "Would more meds help?" is the best they can do.

Gosh, my eating tray needs a Lysol wipe down. I can see crumbs from some other patient's meal. Ew! That huge brown drink cup the nurses left on the tray is fugly in a 1978 Tupperware kind of way. A cleaner scene would sure help me feel better. You know you're in a hospital if the air smells a little bit like pee-pee, with an extra dose of staleness.

Later, much later, I will lose my mind whenever I smell Lysol. It is a reminder of all the bodily trauma in hospitals and labs. Yes, these places and people heal me. But the smell of Lysol triggers my nose to tell my brain I am about to be stung on my chest, or laid out on a cold table. That I have cancer. That cancer may return. That cancer never left. No gracias! And light a match instead of Lysol, would ya?

# CHAPTER 12

## *Stabbing*

Wake me up while I am finally asleep and I will stab you in the eye. Almost.

Sleeping in a hospital bed is a sweaty, druggy mess. I struggle to sleep there. When painkillers and medicine finally kick in, it's off to dreamland I go. Dreams can be wonderful, since I do not have cancer in any of my dreams. My body is covered in bandages and bruises and wounds, and two drains are attached to each breast, to capture the yellow-red ooze. I feel pinches whenever I move.

Yet every nine minutes, I get a cheery "Hello!" from a nurse or staffer, checking on my vitals or catheter, asking me what I want to eat. I love these folks, seriously, doing such hard work. But how I wish I could be knocked out completely for longer so that I would be forced into sleeping. Weren't drugs created for days like these? Ahem, painkiller addiction is a thing. Outside my room, the hallway produces noises of beeps, intercom announcements, and chatter.

One afternoon, Oscar gently touches my arm, and nudges me awake. He stands over my hospital bed and asks, "Are you OK?"

In a low angry voice, I say hotly, "I want to stab you in the eye. WHY did you wake me up? I was sleeping! WHY?!?!" I rant to him, and cry.

I can so easily picture picking up a yellow pencil and putting it into his left eye. All my yellow pencils are back at home. Though that would disrupt my drains and technically I can't lift my arms right now.

Do not wake a sleeping patient. Ever.

## CHAPTER 13

# *Ouch! Blood Tests*

I want to make nice to the phlebotomists as they approach with a giant needle to painfully take two or three vials of blood. In my medical travels, it would shock me when any patient would be rude to the medical staff. I always go for brownie points with anyone taking care of me. Also, I love to schmooze and talk to anyone. Yet, maybe the great juju will help me get better soon? Or maybe being nice is a sure way to keep the staff comfortable and happy while they work on me.

Chat the staff up. Listen to their stories. When it is obvious that the medical pro who is revealing that she's also a confirmed cat lady, I think to myself, "Where's her 'Hang in there' kitten poster?" That would distract me so I can ignore that my arm has been tied off tightly with a thin rubber tube.

I fake-smile when my arm is stabbed fifteen times. I grimace and sweat some as we wait for a trickle. Sometimes I tell the blood takers that I have tiny veins, which is true. But usually they give me a "Duh! I am an expert and already know that" kind of vibe.

Thinking yoga-y thoughts where I am laying down and breathing slowly or fantasizing about chocolate ice cream helps distract me. When all else fails, fantasies about food or sex or food and sex will while away the time. A bribe of chocolate before or after being poked and prodded is a way to make my outing more tasty and fun in keeping with my motto of treating myself to something nice and hopefully free or cheap at least once a day, very important.

Back in my fantasy brain, imagining a gentle oil rubdown from my favorite movie or rock star is ideal. Perhaps while (s)he rubs me down, my star can avoid pressing on my blood-draw consolation prize: a purple and bruised arm that is oh-so-tender.

## CHAPTER 14

# BRCA1 & Angelina Jolie

I send Angelina Jolie a thank you card that I'm sure she put on her fridge, next to drawings from her adorable brood, or beyond-glam travel pics.

On the teensy chance she's reading this, I want to thank Angelina for being so public with the results of her BRCA1 gene test, which revealed a greatly increased risk of breast cancer.

Angie, your acting and love life are interesting enough. But when you had a preventative mastectomy surgery to have your breasts removed, it was heavily covered in the media. Your medical history details and idea to have surgery really stuck with me. So after some back and forth with my hunky husband, I decided to go ahead and get a second opinion when a small pebble under my armpit wouldn't go away. I didn't know where to go. It took me a few weeks to figure out which doctor to visit, who was in network, etc. Medical mazes are common in America, and like many women everywhere, I tend to put my own needs last.

Knowing that you went through the same weird medical testing helps. I got myself through the semi-humiliating procedure of spitting into a shot-size plastic cup for the longest eight minutes. If you can be cool and calm, I can try and do the same when faced with tough medical tests.

Angie, did any of your aunts and cousins ghost you after you messaged them the how-to for BRCA1 testing? What'd you do next, Ang? I know in my heart of hearts that it's best to share info without expecting anything in return. But I am a recovering control freak and want to hear my relatives tell me how fearless and amazing I am for going through so many procedures and complications.

Knowing what you went through helps me feel like I have something in common with you. Minus your long beautiful locks, magazine-worthy posh outfits, properties, and phat bank accounts.

## CHAPTER 15

# *How Going to a Naked Hot Springs Retreat Helped Me Accept My Breast Cancer Surgery Scars*

PUBLISHED IN *Health* MAGAZINE

With cancer, the urge for sex may disappear and cause emotional upheaval. A breast cancer diagnosis at age thirty-nine wrecked me via: seven invasive surgeries, including DIEP (Deep Inferior Epigastric Perforators) flap surgery, where my skin, blood vessels, and fat were removed and transferred from my abdominal tissue (belly fat) to reconstruct new breasts. Because I carry the BRCA1 gene mutation like Angelina Jolie, I opted for a full hysterectomy. With that came insta-menopause, yikes.

My medical dance card also includes sixty-nine blood draws, twenty-two chemotherapy infusions, and eleven infections. Two memorable infections include staph that was transmitted to my wounds when I was in the operating stadium for the DIEP surgery. A later infection to my kidneys was so painful that I hobble-walked to the ER in the middle of the night. Yeast infections and three fierce bouts of the flu demonstrate the fact that although I am out of active treatment, things are far from "all good."

I look normal with my clothes on, but because I don't have a left nipple and my right breast is cleaved in half with a series of angry-looking, red, raised scars, I sometimes feel like Frankenstein. On the left breast, the scarring stems from necrosis, which is dying and rotting flesh. The staph infection forced the surgical team to go in to repair and remove more skin six days after the original DIEP procedure. While my options now include a nipple tattoo or similar cosmetic fix, my interest in being poked and prodded again, even if it promises a "better me," is low.

Because of the way my body looks, I'd been avoiding something that should feel normal: sex with my husband, who I've been with for fifteen years. My experience with sex and breast cancer is hardly unique. Studies show that a wide range of self-reported sexual problems are higher in breast cancer patients versus gynecological or colorectal cancers.

Scars can be emotional as well, says Karen Whitehead, a Georgia-based licensed counselor for women affected by breast cancer: "The scars from breast cancer can affect a woman's sense of sexuality and femininity, self-esteem, sex drive, desire for intimacy, and body image. It is not uncommon for women to feel defective or damaged in some way."

Pre-cancer, marital sex levels were OK. I blame myself because I probably had some undiagnosed depression after my son was born, and the blues come and go. Also, growing up left me feeling disconnected from my body. While I was told as a little girl over and over that I should wait to have sex until I get married, I wasn't sure I ever wanted to get married. I wanted to kiss (and more!) all kinds of people. My early physical urges and crushes became extra confusing, and I didn't have access to pamphlets or books that would help me learn about puberty and otherwise normal physical development.

With my husband, I sometimes pined for more chances to do fun stuff like don a yellow lacy lingerie number. Post-cancer, I seek out ideas in support groups for common issues like lowered sex drive, emotional difficulties, cancer brain (permanent mental fog), eyelash loss, physical weakness, and always feeling like the other shoe will drop and cancer will recur or worsen. Vaginal dryness can be remedied with lots of lube, sure. But my brain too often freezes me up, where I am not able to believe that I am a sexual being. This decrease in desire is striking, and common. A fellow breast cancer patient named Angel Wells, age thirty-four, says, "Not only did breast cancer take one of my breasts, it broke my sexuality. I was completely unprepared for the pain and lack of sex drive, not to mention the strain on my relationship. I feel broken as a woman."

Perhaps it's because I literally can't feel swaths of my chest and tummy. I am furious and sad that having my tubes tied forced me into deciding that I could not or would not try to have another child. Maybe I assume that my awesome spouse somehow views me as broken, ugly and less-than. Relaxing on a comfy couch with the remote control is way easier than addressing my issues.

Other women living with breast cancer share similar experiences. Another patient, AK, age thirty-five, says, "When I was diagnosed, I couldn't even look at my breasts the same way again and I was worried my husband would feel the same. Now that one of them is covered in scars, there's a constant reminder of the cancer that invaded my body. We could maintain a normal sex life through chemo and radiation but the hormone therapy has taken a toll, to say the very least. The almost complete lack of sex drive, weight gain, and awful pain associated with sex now is just unfair. It wasn't supposed to be like this at age thirty-five. Sex can never be spontaneous for us anymore and sometimes that makes me feel like a failure. It sounds harsh, but it's real and something I'm constantly working through. My husband is patient, kind, loving, and exactly the man I expected him to be through all this. We're figuring out this new normal together."

A third patient named Stephany says, "I've been with my husband since I was twenty and I'm forty-two. We've always had a great sex life. Sometimes that's all we had. Once I had my mastectomy and he became my caregiver, things changed for a bit. I had multiple infections, emergency surgeries. He had to sponge-bathe me and hold my hair while I barfed my brains out crying. I had the roughest time with my expanders [a type of breast implant]. I've gained twenty-two pounds. So now I'm doughy with weird tits and no nipples!

"After I got the implants and expanders out, our sex life resumed but not like it was before. I'm *super* self-conscious of my naked chest and refuse to have sex without a top on or a bra. Completely the opposite of how I was before. He's also weird around my boobs, like he's afraid. He tells me he doesn't want to hurt them but I think he's having a harder time than he's letting on. I've never had to think about sex and what I was wearing/going to wear. Totally lame. But cancer is lame."

I wanted to improve my withered sexuality—and two nights at a clothing-optional hot spring seemed like a good next step. In my late twenties, I visited secluded nude beaches a handful of times with a paramour—there were never crowds because we'd visit on weekdays. There, I learned the art of laying a towel on half my body, while I'd let the sun warm my face, arms, chest, and upper body.

The Sierra Hot Springs, in Northern California, is billed as rustic, healing, and sacred. A natural bounty of butterflies, deer, dragonflies, bees, and hummingbirds amid tall trees and summer greenery, it feels worlds away from my normal urban routine of medical appointments, writing, cooking, walking my dog, and carpooling with my nine-year old son.

I spent most of my time at the main Temple dome pool area, with a pool shaded by three large, triangular-shaped beige shading tents overhead.

An outdoor sauna is across from the pool and connected to a building that houses a dry sauna. Seating is available on a shaded wooden deck across from the pool and facing the fields and far off main road with ant-size vehicles going to and from the outside world.

A nearby wooden open-air geodesic dome has a 110-degree hot tub centered under skylights—one sensual feature is the gray sand at the hot tub's bottom, which is a new yet fun experience. By the wall, there are two baby blue cold plunge baths. For more eye candy, colorful rocks dot the mosaic hot tub, and a stained glass window of a mysterious female brunette seems both siren and silent hostess.

The dome has a path leading to the all-gender locker room, where two women don bikini bottoms and go without tops or towels. Everyone else is completely nude. I rush a bit as a newbie to remove the cotton dress I am wearing, as well as my underwear, which I roll up and place into a wooden cubby. In a move straight out of my junior high days, I quickly drape a towel around my trunk so that my vagina and breasts are covered. Mean girls pop up everywhere, right? Better to be on guard at all times.

I walk out and select a deck lounge chair at the end of the row. I'd rather have nature to my right and just one human to my left when I get to the business of lying around in increasing modes of undress. I am naked under my soft gray towel and peek under my giant pink sunglasses to see what the male-to-female ratio is—roughly 50-50. Sunglasses and a big floppy hat are musts, mainly because they enhance my ability to look at others and see if anyone is looking at me. These hot springs couldn't cure my vanity. Without the sunglasses, I avert my gaze and look only at faces within a five-foot radius. My flip-flops are under the lounge chair, and I am lying on another towel—shoulders and legs are fully exposed. I keep rearranging my tote bag in an overly busy fashion—maybe I enjoy this new vacation setup, but I am still not ready to bare more skin. It's not shyness as much as mentally amping myself up to realize that I am just a body here—not more or less, just another paying customer seeking Zen.

I have zero emotional ties to the fifteen or so folks lounging around in various stage of undress, which helps me ease into being fully nude. I'm not sure I'd want to be at the hot springs with friends—and I would not want any men I know (besides my husband, who I left at home) to see my scars. Letting male friends see me nude would inject a too-hot dose of vulnerability into my brain. Plus, I sometimes still feel confused about the guilt and strict mores of my religious upbringing. I'd probably think, "I know what Steve's dick looks like," to myself if my male friends were around.

During my stay, I see that it's easy to eavesdrop on conversations held in *sotto voce*—run of the mill social "How is so and so?" catching up. One couple stays deep in fervent discussion about some ongoing family saga.

It is an odd relief to scope out all the butts, legs, arms, penises, vaginas, and yes, breasts in my sightline, helping me understand that the shapes and forms are diverse—although I do not see anyone lacking a nipple. I also silently award myself a Most Body Scars prize. While I am gratified to see breasts and bodies that aren't thin and taut movie stereotypes, what I hope to see is one surgical scar on other women— maybe at least the slash of a C-section. My Most Body Scars title makes me feel like I should explain the whys behind my scars and revert to my usual chatty self. Sitting still and letting the world face my scars feels tough but needed.

That first hour, I notice how serene and relaxed folks look, as well as the hair grooming norms (natural pubes seem en vogue), which is refreshing.

Later, I home in on one woman in her seventies, gray hair up in a loose bun. I soon think of her as my unofficial elder and guide, even though we never speak. I imagine that she has faced her own challenges and illnesses. A few minutes after observing her, I mimic the way she walks slowly, with a soft smile, from the dome's hot tub to her chair. If she does it, I can too, right? She looks serene in her nudity. I long for the peace that she has.

Being quiet and near water for hours on end is luxurious, but I do also read a book or magazine, pausing to write observations down. I am tired from all the heat—sweating in the steamy wooden sauna, then moving to the pool's water, where I float and bob on my back while my breasts point up and out of the water. The floating is freeing, in part because I always enjoy how soft and serene it is to gaze at the sky while feeling buoyed by a body of water. My body readiness process reminds me of learning to swim in third grade, when I would at first be afraid of the six-foot marker at the community pool; only practice and instilling the memory of how to move my legs and arms while breathing got me closer and closer to feeling safe and comfy.

Later, showering in a private stall, I can smile in the same way as the senior bunned woman. A thin, flowered curtain is all that separates me from two different young women, who greet me by openly smiling and chatting (about the towel hamper). There's a hearty man with his back to us, using the lockers right outside. That's a novelty being so close to naked strangers, and stirs curiosity, and desire. Slowly lathering, as I gaze out the window at a sunny field, I wonder if folks ever pleasure themselves in these showers (a legit question since there is signage throughout forbidding sexual activity of any sort—while cheekily pointing out that rooms are available for just that).

I head back to my spot, still shielding myself from (imagined) glances. I lay a towel down on the wooden deck, which feels warm on my feet. Maybe I can bravely turn over on my back, and let my breasts hang out freely? As I slowly do this, my face feels warm in a semi-embarrassed fashion—like when I first speak in front of a group in public. Squinting through those sunglasses, I realize that no one is looking at me. It's safe to lay my head back to let the sun shine on my skin—scars and all.

## CHAPTER 16

# I Owe HOW Much?
## Sickness & Taxes

Don't fear the bill reaper! I feel like an official grown-up now, because I have a mountain of medical bills. It's easier to file taxes on time for the first time in years instead of organizing and paying off that mountain of scary bills. When I can't sleep at night I'm debating how to pay my bills. Or maybe whether or not disease will return to my body in the near future. Worrying comes easier late at night, and bills are at the top of the list.

Helpful wisdom from my hundreds of hours on the phone with billers and collection agencies: *Never* press zero when on hold to get info about any medical bill. They think you're especially infirm if you are not able to press a button, so sit tight and get a human on the line twenty-two minutes faster. Also, for sanity's sake, put the phone on speaker. That way, you can read about celeb breakups online. See, you really can have it all!

It helps to put off paying things, because after three or six months, the hospital may get tired of waiting and knock off hundreds of dollars from the bill. That said, go ahead and pay your $9.64 blood lab bill before it goes to collections. A collections notice, even if it's for $9.64, can stay on your credit report for seven years, like some scourge or plague. It's mortifying to admit to "forgetting" a $9.64 bill to one's partner.

All my medical fears and nightmares are exposed when I publicly write this plea in May 2017 to a United States congressman on Medium/NewCo Shift:

"Representative Mo Brooks of Alabama, you're essentially voting me off the island and dumping me into a bay of great white sharks, where I will suffer and die in a sad and bloody fashion. Without medicine and treatment for a pre-existing condition called breast cancer, which I was—surprise!—diagnosed with at age thirty-nine, that's what you're doing. I won't be alone as I gasp for air, since so many other folks with common health problems will be isolated, ignored, and left out: from heart issues, to allergies, asthma, diabetes, other forms of cancer, as well as birth defects and strokes, we will not be able to pay our way to survival in America on your watch. When you allow these pre-existing conditions to be penalized, you're making it become far too expensive for this lady.

"I've had seven surgeries, 22 rounds of chemo, 8 infections and 69 blood draws. I wish my time in clinics, hospitals, and pharmacies did not have to be a part of my life, but realize there are so many fellow patients. We come in many colors, shapes, ages (including infants and children), sizes, and personalities and may share the same goal: to feel better.

"By repealing the Affordable Healthcare Act (ACA) and bringing in a medical system that you think favors "good" people over an often sick forty-three year old like me, your vote essentially dictates how long I will live, and how I will live. Even if I will live.

"Since you have the vote, power and TV time, I am listening to you. But I don't like what you're saying and doing, and am offering a perspective that may persuade you to consider other ideas. As well as people that do not look or talk like you, but deserve help and care just the same.

"When you said on CNN yesterday that people who lead good lives don't have to worry about getting and dealing with pre-existing conditions, you're basically telling the world—and patients like me—that I got cancer because I must be bad. Who are you to judge what is good or bad? There is no morality pledge to being American. I've eaten some juicy cheeseburgers and kissed a lot of folks, but I continually work on myself to try and act as kind and friendly as I can to every being I encounter. If you want to paint folks as bad versus good, I'm not sure what other insights and data I can offer to affirm that I deserve to be able to stay in the city I was born in without plotting for a too-grim economic and health future that could happen tomorrow, next week, or soon.

"Your actions and words are a message that my life is not good and has not been good or worthy of help and consideration. It feels like you are putting the fault on me for getting a breast cancer diagnosis that happened to be the same day as back-to-school night for my young son. Tying my illness and pre-existing condition to a notion of goodness is frankly not fair and should not be a legitimate guiding principle for your vote.

"My local breast cancer support group, for women diagnosed before age forty-five, welcomes an average of thirty new members a month. Are we all "bad" people destined for ginormous medical bills? Or no care at all? Do you genuinely think we have each done so many bad things that would cause us to have varying stages of a cancer that attacks our bodies and weakens us? Cancer causes us to cry and worry in the middle of the night over bills and symptoms. Along with the people we love, as we wonder, how many days/weeks/months/years do I have left?

"How will I pay for it all?

"Should we all really listen to the idea of having us move to whatever state to live, work, and seek treatment in? Please mansplain where this state is, because I have many pals who require constant and quality medical help, access, and information on the pills, chemo, radiation, hormone therapy, hot flashes, horrible reactions better left imagined than described, and itchy skin. The awkward and embarrassing waffling between constipation and diarrhea in the same hour is a reality that is a visual and physical reminder of how precarious and crappy one's health is. There's also ongoing anxiety and exhaustion that comes from knowing you may need other costly treatments and surgeries. All to attempt to kill a disease that is attacking your body.

"At forty-three, I'd like to think and hope that I will be able to watch my son graduate from high school. That would be a day that reflects hope, opportunity and hard work, and one that my own family celebrated with me when I graduated at age seventeen.

"Other milestones tempt me daily to keep going. My mom just passed away, at age seventy-five. She had a series of strokes. You would classify her as another one of your "she must not be a good person" pre-existing condition cases. I can't imagine how (if?) the care in nursing homes, hospitals, therapy, clinics, and skilled/assisted living homes (as well as briefly at the home where my parents lived for twenty-five years) would have been managed under your desired system. She could not move or walk on her own. Getting her to move to another state for us pre-existing condition folks frankly would have been impossible.

"I have clogged eye ducts, another ongoing issue from 22 rounds of chemo. It is often tough for me to type and look at my computer. This being modern times, I show up for work, loves (family), friends and community. My eyes atrophied from chemo, so I have dried up eye ducts that are similar to those of an eighty-three-year-old, according to one of the many doctors I see on a regular basis. That means I often have to apply a steroid cream (medicine) to my eyelids and take a lot of time to wash my eyelids daily. That and using warm compresses helps my eyes feel closer to normal, although I do always need to have artificial tears nearby.

"This has all become routine, and involves me regularly going to a doctor and nearby pharmacy, where I sometimes sit on the ground because I am too tired and would not ask a senior or fellow ill person for their chair. A texting teen may get a meaningful gaze from me if I am especially zonked.

"I have brittle bones from going through early menopause. My hysterectomy was tied to a tough decision related to learning through cancer treatment that I carry the BRCA1 gene—another unwanted medical surprise. There are many hours where I can barely stretch or move, because my joints are weak and stiff. That's something I did not experience before I got that call from a lady doctor when I was thirty-nine. I am a good enough person, but instead got dealt a tough or less than ideal break genetically and medically speaking.

"Again, why should my innate goodness matter?

"Environmental factors are also at play when it comes to the causes of breast cancer, but my words here are meant to keep the focus on who deserves health care and why.

"I have volunteered to help others since I could walk as a toddler. Although my younger brother would probably have called it "bossiness" over "help." I am friendly and enthusiastic often. When I see someone that needs a hand—from getting donations for a fundraiser for science labs at my son's school to carrying groceries or offering an ear or advice to a fellow patient or writer who may be younger or older than me, I give it. I will carry someone's books or bags if they look like they are in worse shape than me. Even though I do tend to get winded or worn out often.

"Congressman, you have the power to make life healthy and good for many of us Americans. I will be watching through my sometimes-cloudy eyes to see what you say and do next. I hope you listen to your constituents, sisters, and friends who may in fact be dealing with pre-existing conditions, extreme worry, serious illness, and disease."

## CHAPTER 17

---

# *Mealtrain Forces Me to Say "Hey" in My Robe*

Getting a Mealtrain means comfort food from friends is delivered at home. Even if I feel weird and hesitant about showing people who care about me what I look like without eyebrows and greet them in my bathrobe because it's midafternoon and I am tired as hell. It's ideal to use an online tool like Mealtrain where I can request help with rides, chores, and email information to answer the annoyingly difficult-to-answer question of "How are you?"

Saying yes to help via Mealtrain is tough, but the great food helps me get out of my own worried head. Remember: the effects of this illness go on and on, and picking an end date is futile. Veggie soup with crusty bread, stuffed-crust pizza, roasted chicken, veggie dal and black bean soup? Yes please. The urge to tidy and dust runs strong on a day when food is delivered, but I remind myself that I don't have the strength to walk up a flight of stairs or make "real" food for myself, so that dusting can wait. It's also easy to fantasize about ooey-gooey pizza or roast chicken on days when I feel sad and mad about being so sick. Having a calendar filled with meals is better than one that only lists enemas, medical appointments, and bill due dates.

## *Home*

Giving myself permission to watch bad TV takes many weeks, and emails from friends who have also had terrible illness nudge me to understand that it's OK to take it easy. Resting should be like a job and the main thing to focus on. Leave that to-do list for much later, or ditch it completely, they say.

When I am drugged or just overly tired, a campy sci-fi series on Net-flix is compelling, and I adore seeing humans turn into werewolves, especially because it means a lot of attractive flesh is on display, and people take their shirts off. Maybe I can't have sex easily with anyone, including myself, but it's nice to feel the kind of desire that is a part of normal everyday life. Adding to the wistful mood, I tend to gravitate toward actors with blue eyes, in part because it stokes memories of a long-ago first love.

On some afternoons, Cipriano gets to watch *a lot* of TV sitting next to me in bed. Some of my best dozing sessions happen while he watches hours of cartoons. If I feel especially comfy, I may even suggest that we eat popcorn in bed, even though finding kernels later is a tad gross and buttery in a bright orangey kind of way.

One day, when I remember that we have an air mattress borrowed from my parents, I have Oscar pump the mattress up and throw a sheet on it so that Cipriano and I can have a slumber party on the floor. I have to squash thoughts of feeling poor; instead go with "Why not?" as a reason to feel like we can still have fun even if Mommy is a zombie. As I lay on the air mattress and note how petite our apartment is and that it could really use a paint job, I can feel happy that there is time for me to rest and let my eyes glaze over while another episode of *Scooby Doo* streams.

CHAPTER 18

---

# *Cuddle Me: Slippers & Robes*

Slippers, robes, and cuddly blankets are musts for a cheesy sex romp in the movies, but sickies need them, too. When I am gifted fuzzy and cozy items (robe, velour tracksuit, slippers, scarves), it means that I can get winks of sleep and slivers of relaxation. My new cozy goods acknowledge the obvious fact that my activities are limited to walking to and from the bathroom, and moving from the bathroom to my super couch or bed, to lay around and look at celebrity magazines or, on an ideal day, to rest and nap. One of the toughest parts about being ill is letting myself feel it's OK to snooze, even a little. Relaxing is a new concept to me, because I am not comfortable sitting around without checking off items on a too-long to-do list.

With so much pain and so many bills to worry about, the gift givers are doing for me what I can't afford to do for myself. These gifty items definitely feel like a special treat. If someone asks me "What can I do for you?" it would never cross my mind to ask for a cozy robe. But when I receive a gift, it feels so nice, because my budget and energy remain focused on saving up to pay my medical bills.

Some gifts come as a total surprise. A prayer blanket touches my heart and helps keep my feet and hands warm—with chemo, I am cold deep in my bones often. How nice that it is in two cooling shades of gray, which just happens to match the peeling paint of my apartment's living room. I am not religious and identify as a spiritual hippie but appreciate the idea of people knitting and crafting something for me. Think about the process: after they knit, they probably stand together as a group and pray over the blanket. I've always loved being the center of attention as well as crafts done by other talented folks. Let those worlds collide! With the prayer blanket, these kind humans give me strength when I am suffering from insomnia, restlessness, sadness, and overall exhaustion.

# CHAPTER 19

## *The New Normal*

My consolation prize after all my surgeries and treatments is the body of a fit teenager. Hey, I worked hard for this body! Infections and ailments become the new normal. I nickname my eyes "porno eyes," because whenever I look in the mirror in the bathroom, my eyes and lashes have a white-yellow crust.

The discomfort of having ongoing problems frustrates me the most when I try to manage a timeline of some sort—like hey, by this date and this procedure or appointment, I will be 100 percent finished with disease and illness. The new normal is that, actually, my eyes, body, and brain are decimated, and being a little bit sick and definitely prone to infection will be the standard for me until who knows when.

I gross out my nurse-husband and pretend I made fermented coffee gravy with my very own body. So *that's* what infection smells like. When a friend asks why I didn't call the surgeon at the first sign of stink, I don't know what to say. I wanted the surgery to be over, and didn't want to have to go back to the hospital. The infection is so deep that my favorite surgeon will have to operate again, and slice off a nipple that has necrosis (a fancy word that means the nipple skin has died). My own flesh has died on the vine, and it looks yellow and gray. I cope with all this ooze by joking about it with my son, while I try in my head to not beat myself up too much about waiting to report the smelly symptoms to the Doc.

## CHAPTER 20

---

# *A Look Back*

I t's now been more than three years since my diagnosis. My last surgery was two years ago. It's been four months since my last wince-inducing blood draw on those damn small veins of mine. I even eventually grumpily realized that the hots for my surgeon had cooled, which gives space for the next patient to get their crush on. Sure, I've been through medical hell—it still shows up in various infections, rashes, and creaky postmenopausal joints.

Spending time with other cancer folks at parades, fundraisers, dance parties, retreats, and support group meetings gives me the chance to be with people who fully understand what I've been through and what my daily life is like now.

It can feel terribly sad when someone has a recurrence or a new death is announced to our group. I completely spiral and go into a grief-stricken daze when the person who died was someone I really got to know. Yet, these deaths also deepen my urge to do more. Because yup, cancer still sucks, and no amount of my favorite bright gold eyeshadow or awesome looking thrift store accessories can ever change that.

# *Acknowledgements*

Illustrator Don Asmussen partnered with me on this project because he always makes me laugh and knows what it's like to be bald and in pain from his own semi-terrible cancer journey. Don's comedic visuals are at turns laugh-out-loud funny and poignant.

Without Regan McMahon's eagle-eyed edits, I would keep confusing the words grey/gray, as well as blonde/blond, and make related type-written mistakes. She brings terrific professional copyediting skills along with smarts and kindness. I love having her help and friendship.

Since Josh Korwin works on the award-winning ZYZZYVA literary journal (ahem!), it is amazing to have him transform my words and Don's funny illustrations into something beautiful.

When I am crying, mad or sad with snot running down my face, I try to get over it or at least remember how much help I've gotten:

**DOCTORS**

Dr. Evangeline Amores, Dr. Gabriel Kind, Dr. Gauri Kelekar, Dr. Kevin Knopf, Dr. Nima Grissom.

**NIPPLE TATTOO ARTIST**

Cathi Locati of Final Mile Ink.

# ACKNOWLEDGEMENTS

## COMMUNITY

Adriano Hrvatin, Amy Callaway, April McGill, Barbara Denson, Barbara Meacham, Ben Alamar, Beth Harris, Blair Jackson, Bob Blum, Bobbers Ladd, Carrie Sullivan, Carmen Jacinto Sandoval, Catalina Chavez, Celia Barbaccia, Chandra Egan, Christie Ward, Christine Garofoli, Claudia Villalon, Claudine Asbaugh, Cliff Lee, Cory Ladd, Cristina Johnson Polk, Dain Whiting, Dana Van Gorder, David Serrano, DeeDee Serrano, Demetri Rizos, Denise Greig, Dianna Rose, Dominique Serrano, Don Ladd, Dorothy Whittenburg, Emily Mariko-Sanders, Emma Bailey, Eric Sloan, Erica Engin, Erin Neeley Archuleta, Gabrielle Whiting, Gayla Selinger, Grace Degnan, Gretchen Ladd, Henry Lucero, Howard Moorin, Irene Blum, Jeff Sprague, Jen Craft, Jeri Hagen, Jerry Garchik, Jessica Wright, Joe Sandoval, John Caldwell, John Memminger, Josh Chisom, Josh Ladd, Josue Hurtado, Julie Tan, Justine Janney, Kate Sherwood, Kathryn Poole Cohen, Kelly Ladd Whiting, Ken Nelson, Kim Teevan, Kirsten Macintyre, Kiwi Whiting, Leslie Kaye, Lisa Rogovin, Liza Ladd Bledsoe, Lora Blum, Malea Chavez, Marc Puich, Mark Bethel, Mary Ann Ladd, Matthew Harris, Mary Beth Maloney, Mike Bledsoe, Mindy Chroust Davenport, Monica Meinardi, Nicole Murgia, Nick Murgia, Nick Pagoulatos, Oscar D. Villalon (Suegro), Pam Dawkins Lazatin, Paul Dally, Patricia DeFonte, Patty Rhee, Philip Walker, Robert Moon, Roy Salazar, Sandra Huerta, Sarah Davis, Scott Degnan, Shanagh Dely, Shawn Lytle, Stacy Beugen, Stephanie Nix, Steve Cooper, Steve Hagen, Steve Villalon, Sue Wagerman Gibbs, Tasan Engin, Yogesh Sharma.

## AUTHORS, BOOKSELLERS, CREATIVES, EDITORS, PUBLISHERS & WRITERS

Alia Volz, Alphonso Montouri, Althea Wasow, Amy Alamar, Amy Sherman, Andrew Tonkovich, Barbara Berman, Brett Hall Jones, Byron Spooner, Caridwen Irvine-Spatz, Carter Taylor Seaton, Christian

Berthelsen, Christopher Cook, Christin Evans, Daniel Handler, David R. Baker, David Corbett, David Ulin, Delfin Vigil, Eddie Muller, Ethan Watters, Elise Proulx, Garrett Law, Glen David Gold, Gregory Spatz, Heidi Benson, Jack Boulware, Jane Ganahl, Jason Roberts, Jen Leo, Joal Ryan, Joe Garofoli, Joe Shoulak, Joel Riddell, Joel Selvin, John Freeman, John McMurtrie, Josh McHugh, Judith Bernard, Julia Scheeres, Julia Scott, Julia Wackenheim, Julie Lindow, Kate MacMillan, Kelly Zito, Kevin Hunsanger, Kevin Smokler, Kitty Margolis, Laura Cogan, Laura Fraser, Laura Howard, Lea Mahan, Leah Garchik, Lee Sherman, Leonardo, Leslie Berriman, Leticia Hernández-Linares, Lisa Alvarez, Lisa Brown, Lisa Hix, Louis B. Jones, Marcia Gagliardi, Meredith White, Marge Pearson, Nancy Hayes, Nion McEvoy, Paul Aleman Jr., Paul Hubler, Paul Beatty, Paul Yamazaki, Peter Hartlaub, Peter Lawrence Kane, Peter Maravelis, Peter Orner, Peter White, Pia Sarkar, Robert Mailer Anderson, Roberto Lovato, Sam Barry, Sands Hall, Scott M. Gimple, Sean Timberlake, Seth Rosenfeld, Stephanie Rosenbaum Klassen, Stephen Bertram, Steve Chen, Steve Gibbs, Steve Ryfle, Susan Ito, Tamara Palmer, Ted Weinstein, Teresa Moore, Tom Barbash, Tyson Law, Vanessa Hua.

### ORGANIZATIONS

Alanon, Bay Area Young Survivors (BAYS), Breast Cancer Action (BCA), Commonweal, Community of Writers at Squaw Valley, Gibson, Dunn & Crutcher LLP; Litquake, San Francisco Tenants Union, We Wai Kai Nation, The Writers Grotto and ZYZZYVA.